Copyright © 2023 LAUREN GANIM

All rights reserved.

ISBN: 9798335723725

DEDICATION

This book is dedicated to every person who has ever felt inadequate due to health reasons beyond their control. This work was born from the compassion for the many thoughtful, kind & generous people I met along my journey, as well as for myself. The journey back to health & self-love is something that I wish for every person who picks up this book. The fight for my family was hard won, and my three beautiful children, Maron, Paul & Gabriel, are testaments to the power of a mother's love and a father's strength. This work is dedicated in their honor. Thank you for choosing me to be your mother; it is the privilege of a lifetime.

Contents

ACKNOWLEDGMENTS

This book could not have been possible without the unwavering support of my mother, Martha Fulcher. Her deep expertise in the fields of Reproductive Endocrinology, Obstetrics & Gynecology as well as her compassion & support, made her an invaluable partner throughout every single part of this journey. My husband, AJ, for his constant love & support. Sarah Gross, Anne Kinchin, Dr. Pickens A. Gantt & Dr. Norbert Gleicher all lent their time & expertise to my journey and left an indelible mark on my family & my heart. Finally, this book would not have been possible without the great love, vision & sacrifice of my father, Dr. Paul Howard Fulcher, Jr., who dedicated his life to the health of women & children.

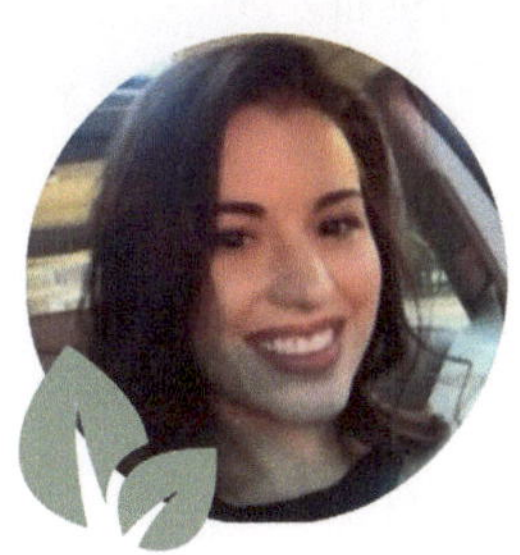

I.   Introduction:

My name is Lauren Ganim and I am the mama to three pretty incredible kids. I'm also a professional marketer for a Fortune 500 company, and the daughter of an Obstetrician/Gynecologist & a nurse with a certification in Reproductive Endocrinology Nursing. I also have a deep passion to help fellow would-be mamas who are struggling to conceive, as I once did. It took me 5 years and $50,000 to conceive my first child, and the scars from infertility still run deep. But they are nothing compared to the joy my family brings me, which is how this project was born. I'm lucky that throughout my journey, I had resources that many women do not. In the spirit of sisterhood and paying it forward, I want to be here for you - like an older sister or a best friend that has been through it & seen it all.

Studies show that women struggling with infertility have just as high of levels of anxiety and depression as those with terminal cancer diagnoses. And it's no wonder...infertility robs you of so much. It's like a death sentence. It robs you of joy in your relationships, life loses its meaning- when you are lost in the woods of infertility, it seems like you will never get out. I will never forget sitting in the office of the Director of the Fertility Clinic at Cleveland Clinic, and her telling me to "stop wasting my money" on IVF treatments and to go find a surrogate. I cried the whole way home, with my husband awkwardly trying to comfort me from the driver's seat.

Since my discovery on how to heal myself & conceive, I have developed a deep passion to help fellow would-be mamas. Supporting women throughout this process is my mission and the driving purpose of my life. Because here's the thing: unfortunately, Reproductive Endocrinology is a business. It's a game of numbers, and although helping women should be of the highest order, capitalism creeps in. It is essential that you become the biggest advocate for your own health- it shouldn't have to be that way, but here we are. If you want to be a mother (or a father), and you have the drive and tenacity to be your own advocate & educator throughout this process,

YOU WILL SUCCEED. It doesn't matter who told you no. It doesn't matter how old you are. If you truly in your heart want to be a parent, you will. The path forward may not always look like you thought it would, but at the end of it, you will still have a beautiful child in your arms. Ultimately this plan- along with the dozens of other resources and guides I've shared- reflects at the heart what I'm motivated to do every single day: to serve fellow women and celebrate the amazing ability we have (yes, YOU!) to usher life into this world. Take heart, mama. Help is on the way.

A word about inclusivity: Throughout this book, I refer to 'you' or 'motherhood' as I am a cis heterosexual female and I am speaking from my experience and point of view. However, the advice contained in this book should be helpful for men seeking to boost fertility as well as non-binary members of the LGBTQ community (and if this is you, I'm working on something special just for you!). Wherever possible, I will refer to 'parenthood' as opposed to 'motherhood,' however, many of the medical interventions described in this book relate to female anatomy. As an American, my experience is with the healthcare system within the United States and thus my experience is with the healthcare system & insurance policies in the United States.

"My hope is that this will be an empowering resource
that fills some very big holes currently out there
about infertility and reproductive endocrinology"

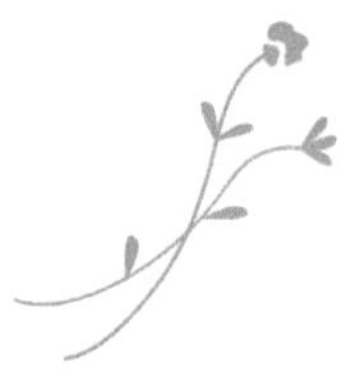

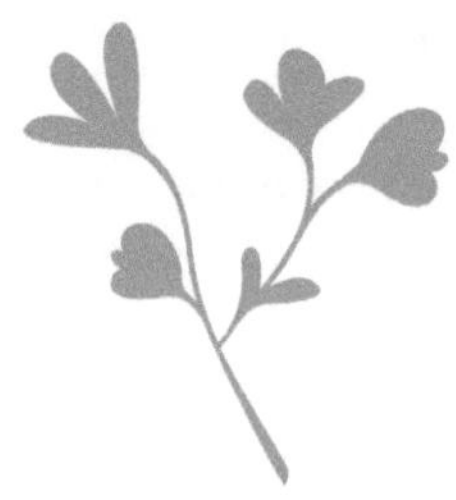

II.   Open Arms, Aching Heart: My Story

Approximately 10% or 6.1 million women in the United States experience infertility (defined as either difficulty in getting or staying pregnant). Ladies, that's a lot of us. And it's not something many people talk about openly. It's stigmatized- maybe you feel like it's your "fault." Maybe you blame your partner. Maybe you secretly hate your friends/colleagues/that high school kid who got pregnant without any troubles. You find it difficult to be in social settings. Seeing family turns from a refuge to an indeterminable barrage of questions 'so, when are you guys having kids?' I get it. I've been there. Oh, was I ever there.

You see, I thought I was smart. Being the daughter of an OB/GYN, I was brought up with a lot of medical information- way more than my peers. In high school, I was the kid everyone asked for sex-ed advice; my parents were guest speakers at the school on the topic! After I went away to college, I promptly began the Pill, and stayed on it over ten years, thinking nothing of the consequences (they weren't really known then anyway). I met my husband in college, but we didn't get married for 8 years as we were both establishing our careers, traveling, and enjoying young adult life in the city. I never considered that I would have trouble conceiving, even though the early signs were there.

What signs? Well, for many years I struggled with an eating disorder, which eventually caused amenorrhea (irregular or periods that completely stop). In truth, I never had regular periods, as my ED began prior to menstruation. I would bleed for 3 days, once a year. While I knew this was not healthy, I considered myself "lucky" that I didn't have to deal with the monthly cramps my girlfriends complained of and figured that as soon as I started eating properly, my periods would regulate. And although I was thin, I also dealt with constant inflammation, which could be seen in my distended "pot belly" and fed my eating disorder even more. Brain fog, cramping & constipation I all considered a way of life. I thought constant stomach pains were normal, and that everyone else obviously just dealt with them better than me; that I must be a 'whiner' or a wimp.

After we got married and decide to try to have children, I went off the pill and for over a year nothing happened. My periods went from sporadic to non-existent once I was not on the pill. Frustrated, we tried Clomid several times, however, my ovaries became so polycystic we could never complete a cycle. This was the first piece of alarming medical diagnosis I had ever received- I had Polycystic Ovarian Syndrome (PCOS). I was confused. How could I have PCOS? True, I didn't get periods like other women, but weren't PCOS women obese? I was slim. Didn't PCOS women have mustaches? I didn't have facial hair or any of the outward markers that would normally cause a physician to look for PCOS, which is how it had been missed for so long.

It was around this time that I became determined to conquer my eating disorder for good. Although I was much better than I had been in my teens, old habits were hard to break when in times of intense stress or depression. As I worked to normalize my nutrition, I began to notice problems with my digestion. Food would sit in my stomach like a rock (one reason, I realized, that I had such a strong impulse to throw it up). My digestion was such an issue that at 28 years old, I had a colonoscopy and a defecography. It was painful and humiliating as well as fruitless; I was not taken seriously and was given a diagnosis of Irritable Bowel Syndrome (IBS) and sent on my way. During this time, I specifically inquired if I might have something more serious, like Crohn's or celiac disease and was told no. It was many years later that I was diagnosed with Celiac Disease and learned that I was never even checked for celiac during these procedures, even though I had the invasive procedures necessary to determine a diagnosis and had specifically asked. Surprise, surprise, a young female's complaints not being taken seriously.

My doctors recommended In Vitro Fertilization (IVF) as a next step, given that Clomid wasn't working. This sent me into an emotional tailspin. I didn't WANT to conceive this way. What if I spent all this time and money and it didn't work? Even worse, I knew that the process of IVF, as emotionally draining as it is, would COMMIT me to this label of 'infertile.' I would be an infertile woman, and when it didn't work, I would be devastated. It was a huge emotional and financial risk, and I was terrified that my heart would never heal from it. Eventually, though, I rallied my courage for the good of my unborn children, and we began IVF at the Cleveland Clinic. Devastatingly, we never were able to fully complete a cycle. My polycystic ovaries were at it once again, ruining any chance I had of insemination. I was told that I would never conceive, that I was wasting my money and time; given a pamphlet on surrogacy & sent on my way. I cried for months.

Laid completely bare, I hit bottom. I felt guilty that I was "depriving" my husband of the children he wanted so badly. I imagined that he wanted to divorce me. I considered leaving him for "his own good." To say it was a dark time is an understatement. Exhausted from the constant poking and prodding, I told the hubs that I needed a break. We booked a trip to Europe in the hopes of rejuvenation, and perhaps to prove to ourselves that our lives could still have meaning without children. On that trip we encountered multiple families with adopted children, and my husband implored me to stop prostrating myself and sign up for adoption. Although I began reaching out to some adoption agencies, some part of me knew that I wasn't ready to give up yet.

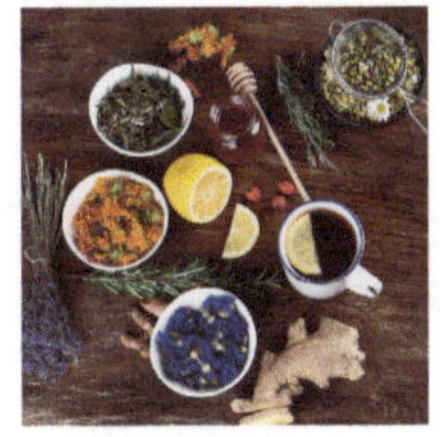

Back at home, I knew that the traditional routes weren't working. I had to do something different, so I turned to ancient remedies via traditional Chinese medicine and Ayurvedic techniques- castor oil packs, acupuncture, teas, tinctures, enough vitamins to choke a horse, massage, meditation, therapy, and a complete overhaul of my diet- everything 100% organic, no plastic or canned food containers. I threw out all my makeup and skincare in favor of holistic options. It was incredibly expensive, but I felt compelled to leave no stone unturned.

Back in the States, my mother (a reproductive endocrinology nurse) told me of a clinical trial she had just read about. The Center for Human Reproduction in NYC with Dr. Norbert Gleicher were doing to assist women with thin uterine lining (only part of my issue). I was game and made an appointment. It was expensive- $400 for a phone consultation, and approximately $25,000 in lab work, as Dr Gleicher turned over every stone. I learned that in addition to Celiac Disease, I had a genetic mutation called MTHFR that inhibited my body from absorbing folic acid (an essential nutrient for fetal brain development) as well as the Fragile X gene, something other centers weren't even aware of as a factor that influences treatment plans and prognoses. I immediately began augmenting my diet and vitamin regimen. Although Dr Gleicher had accepted me for his clinical trial, he suggested we try an innovative hormone therapy first. With all of my previous IF treatments, the focus had been on increasing estrogen, which left me with brain fog, irritability, and generally feeling 'not like myself.' Given my PCOS, Dr Gleicher assessed that although my testosterone levels were higher than average, all of this therapy had reduced them to lower than optimal levels for my particular body. I immediately began testosterone therapy, and within 3 months, normal periods resumed. I was pregnant within a month after that ON MY OWN with no insemination or other intervention. For my second child, we already knew the magic formula, and although this time it took 6 months, I got pregnant on my own again. After my second child, I experienced regular 30-day cycles for the first time in my life, and WITHOUT EVEN TRYING found myself pregnant with our 3rd child- who me, with a surprise baby?! We now have a healthy, thriving family of 5, of which I will never stop being endlessly grateful for. But I also realize that without the advantages I had and without the hard-won education on my personal medical history, my children would not be here.

The science of reproductive endocrinology has come a long way, but patient advocacy (and particularly for the LGBTQ set) has a significant way to go. It is critical that you educate yourself, become your own advocate and learn all you can - do not take no for an answer. You also must take responsibility for what you can control- your diet, your body, and your overall health & wellness regime. Although Western medicine does not tend to focus on these things, we know that they play an important role in conception. Without a multi-pronged approach to health and wellness, conception would not have been possible for me. Although harrowing, I am so glad that I had this experience and now get to share this knowledge with you.

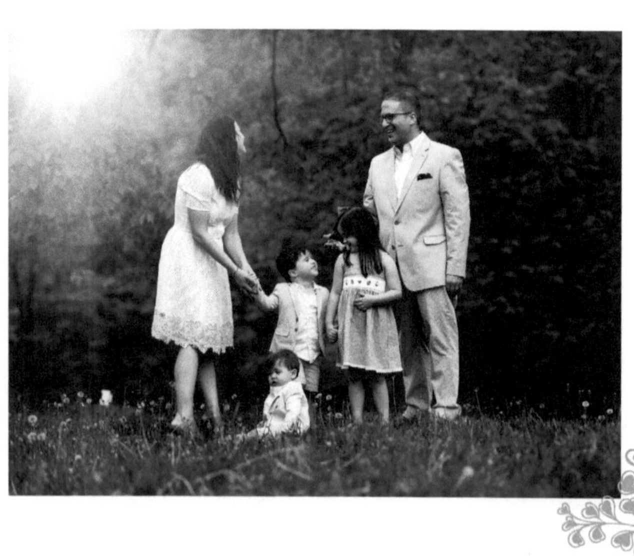

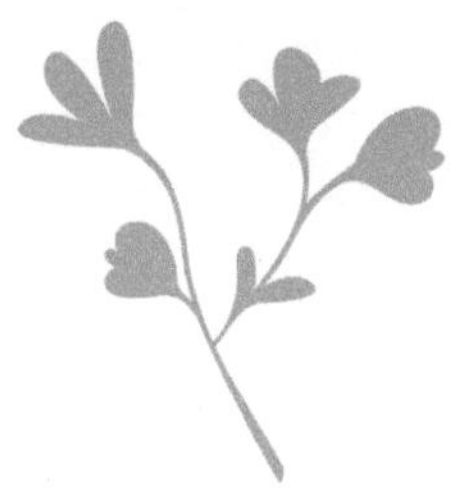

III.   Fertility is a Business.

When medical professionals decide on their career path, the path is laid with good intentions. Most want to help people and regard the Hippocratic oath as a solemn vow. Somewhere along the way, however, capitalism creeps in. Between the insurance companies, the competition for patients, and confusing medical billing, reproductive endocrinology centers are incentivized to make clinic numbers look as favorable as possible: out of X many cases, Y resulted in a successful pregnancy. The clinic with the best figures wins- more patients, more funding, better financial results for the clinic and RE professionals. The unfortunate part of all of this is that patients with the most challenging cases then become discouraged from trying again, so as to limit the impact to clinic numbers. When I finally understood this, it was revolutionary for me. I never considered that my chances of conceiving were being commandeered by the business of infertility. This is why, even though I was physically able to carry and bear three beautiful children into the world, I was actively discouraged from doing so, because my case was a bit more challenging.

Once you understand that there are certain protocols, and if you don't fit into those protocols you will likely be discouraged or turned away, it makes a world of difference. Understand that there may be nothing prohibitive about your biology, just a system that is based on speed, capitalism, and efficiency. This makes it even more important that you understand your specific situation & find healthcare practitioner that works FOR YOU.

Another big mistake a lot of women make is relying on their gynecologist to be aggressive about their infertility- many women unknowingly make this mistake and waste months and years (while precious eggs/fertility is declining) before they take more aggressive steps. A gynecologist may be the first physician that a woman speaks to about her infertility, but gynecologists are not experts in fertility. Some are more informed than others, but most GYNs won't even check an AMH level to see what the ovarian reserve levels are, and many aren't performing regular ultrasounds during treatment with Clomid, so they won't even know if the female was ovulating during the cycle. Additionally, gynecologists have no financial incentive to send a woman to another provider who could do more for her- it is in their financial interest that you keep coming back after each unsuccessful attempt. I'm not saying doctors are bad people- I come from a family of them! - I'm just saying you need to understand how the game is played.

And don't be frustrated with your doctor-he or she isn't trying to thwart your chances of conception; they are simply operating within a framework. Sure, for you, the would-be parent with a broken heart over several failed rounds of Clomid, it would be easier on your heart if you knew up front it wasn't going to work because the bloodwork would have told you about X or Y thing. But spending $20-30K on lab work for every patient isn't reasonable and it's not something most people or our healthcare system in the United States can bear. In medical school, they teach physicians to leverage the protocols that work for most of the population first. Clomid works for most women. So does IVF. If you fall outside of these ranges, just know that you still have options and that you need to get more aggressive quickly. Be frank with your physician and find a team that will work hard for you.

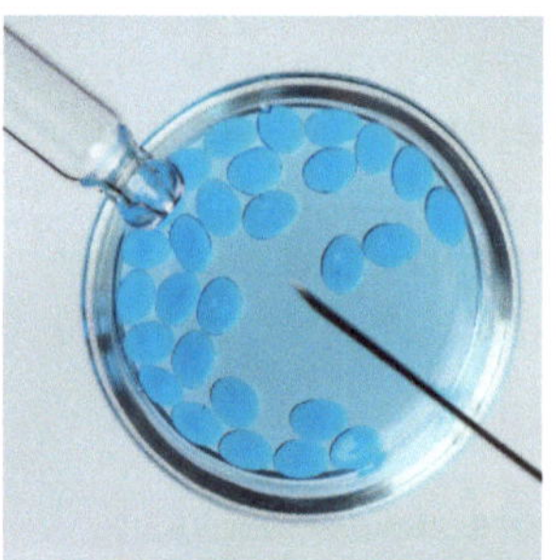

Known as the trend of individualized medicine, we now know that individual biology and DNA can necessitate care plans that are individualized to the patient. If you've gone to a RE clinic and been turned away, take heart. Almost 100% of the women I befriended throughout my IF journey that were struggling as well now have healthy, happy families. Just because you were told 'no' once before doesn't mean you should take it as gospel. In fact, it should fire you up to make your dreams of a family a reality!

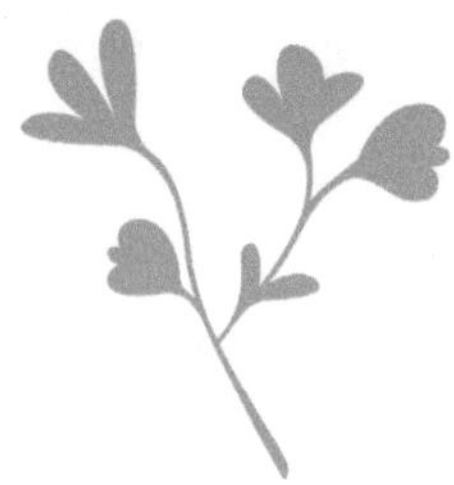

IV.   Commit to Leaving No Stone Unturned

When you are in the weeds of infertility, even the smallest of tasks feels monumental. Every dollar sunk into conceiving, every disappointment, every strained relationship all adds up to something that seems too great to bear. And if you've given it your best shot and still come up empty, there is no shame in charting an alternate course whether that be adoption, surrogacy, or something else entirely-only you know what is best for you. But as I've stated, there is no one else out there looking after your best interests the way YOU will. True, there are some infertility concierge services out there, but they are likely cost prohibitive for most people and still not widely available. Your best bet is to use your own knowledge, resources and burning desire to advocate for yourself. Ask to see your labs, get copies of everything, and develop an at home medical file of your own, so that when and if you need to change providers you can provide accurate information without waiting for medical records to transfer (and sometimes, there are additional fees for doing so). Brush up on your medical records before every appointment so when they ask you what your last TSH level was, you can answer confidently. Keep getting tested and retested, and if your doctor doesn't think you should, change doctors. Bring up bits of information that have been previously ignored- I can't tell you how many providers told me my MTHFR genetic mutation was 'not a big deal.' However, had I not continued to remind my medical team, I would not have known to take METHYLATED FOLATE as opposed to folic acid, as is regularly prescribed to expecting mothers, and likely would have ended up with a child with neural tube defects. This is because the MTHFR genetic mutation is not widely discussed or taught in medical schools- this, however, does not mean it does not have an impact on fetal development. RE is a rapidly evolving field, and while there are protocols that work for most patients, there are new clinical trials and procedures being discovered every day. Get yourself aligned with a healthcare team that pushes boundaries, not just reports success cases on tried-and-true procedures. And while you're at it, build your own infertility team, comprised not only of your Reproductive Endocrinologist and nurses, but your holistic practitioners as well. My team consisted of my acupuncturist, masseuse, family, friends, energy healer, doula, etc. Ask questions and take knowledge from each of these resources to build a care plan that makes sense for you.

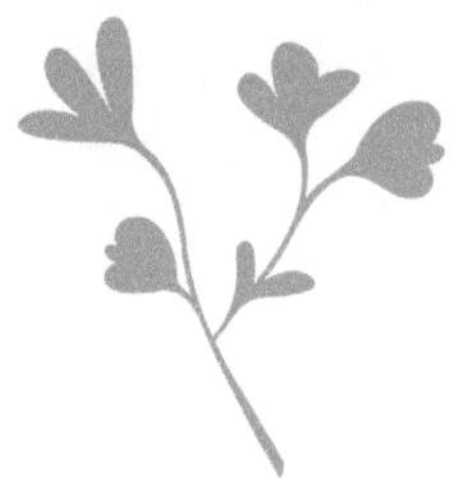

V.   Infertility 101

So, first of all, what is Infertility?
The World Health Organization, physicians and insurance companies all have
a different definition for infertility, but the most broadly accepted definition
is, "the inability to achieve a pregnancy within 1 (or 2) years." This sounds
basic, but it's important, because your definition of infertility might be very
different based on your age, medical history, and personal situation. The 20-
year-old newlywed who didn't get pregnant this year has more options than
the 40-year-old with an autoimmune disorder and a partner with poor
semen analysis. The biggest sin we see with healthcare practioners is
wasting time. Maybe you go to your gynecologist seeking help for infertility.
They take you off contraceptives, make you wait a requisite amount of time
(6 months-1 yr.), maybe they give you some medication (all the while not
checking with regular ultrasounds to see if you are ovulating). It doesn't
work, you get frustrated and lose hope, and worse, you've lost TIME. By the
time a woman is 38-40 years old, fertility is declining RAPIDLY. For me, I was
barely 30 years old, but my PCOS was causing my eggs to age prematurely;
my eggs looked like those of a women ten years my senior! Even the loss of
a few months can be detrimental to success with conception. If you take
anything away from this book, DON'T WAIT for your doctor to get serious.

Ok, so I've been diagnosed as "infertile." Now what?
Well, the first step is an evaluation. Recall from your high school biology
class that in its most basic form, we need sperm, an egg, and a way for them
to come together to create an embryo. Your healthcare practitioner will run
bloodwork on you to test ovarian function & reserve, check for any issues in
the fallopian tubes and likely do a semen analysis on your partner.

When you meet with your physician, get ready to give them the date of the
first day of your last period, the last time you were intimate with your
partner, what methods of contraception you've used in the past, your full
medical history and what you had for breakfast on Tuesday (ok just kidding

about the last one. Kinda). You'll need to quickly get comfortable giving your RE as much information as you have (and again, if you have copies of your medical records, it's always good to bring those to reference). Your RE needs to understand first and foremost, if you are having regular menstrual cycles. If so, are you actually ovulating during those cycles? If not, you need to figure out why. If you ARE ovulating, then we need to look at things like sperm quality, egg quality and your uterus. Maybe your uterine lining is not thick enough to "hold" onto a fertilized egg. Maybe you have another abnormality in your uterus, or a clotting disorder that could cause issues. All of this needs to be considered to obtain a diagnosis to work against. Your goal right now should be to get a diagnosis. Without that, you can't move forward. "I'm just not pregnant" is no longer good enough- let's get serious!

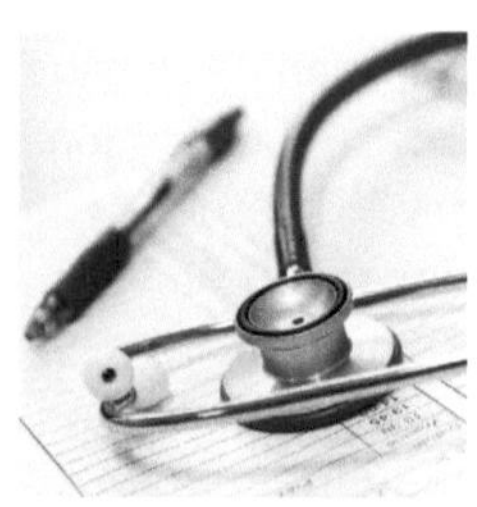

Part of the basic workup also typically includes a Hysterosalpingogram (HSG). This procedure looks at the basic shape of the inside of your uterus- maybe you have a tilted uterus or some other uncommon condition that's not been previously identified. In HSG, a thin tube is threaded through the vagina and cervix. A substance known as contrast material is injected into the uterus. A series of X-rays, or fluoroscopy, follows the dye, which appears white on X-ray, as it moves into the uterus and then into the tubes. If there is an abnormality in the shape of the uterus, it will be outlined. If the tube is open, the dye gradually fills it. The dye spills into the pelvic cavity, where the body reabsorbs it. I will also add that while uncomfortable, this procedure is not painful for most people.

Next, you will need to understand if your ovaries are functioning appropriately. Some doctors will test your estradiol, but you must take this test on a specific day in your cycle, which can be difficult, if like me, you don't know what cycle day you are on because your cycles are erratic. Another way to test for this is by looking at your AMH (anti-Mullerian hormone) levels, and this blood test can be drawn at any time. Think of this as your "egg count" test- within a week, your physician will have a highly predictive marker for your ovarian function. Higher AMH values (greater than 1 ng/mL) usually signify that a woman has a normal ovarian reserve and lower numbers (less than 1 ng/mL) may indicate a woman with a low or diminished ovarian reserve (known as DOR). We know that a woman's fertility declines as she ages so typically, we see AMH values also start to decline as women age. The value of this test is that a woman with a low AMH can choose to do something about her fertility now if she desires a family for the future. Again, this will vary by center and physician; some doctors will say that if you have an AMH of less than 2 you have a problem, while other physicians maintain that 2-4 is a healthy & acceptable range. If your RE clinic is one of the ones that use tried and true protocols, and they aren't open to innovative technologies & procedures, many won't take on a patient with an AMH of less than 2. But don't despair if you get turned down by a clinic due to a low AMH number- you can change it through medications and changes in lifestyle. For me with my PCOS, my AMH was off the charts (30)- meaning I had a ton of eggs but given PCOS none of them could grow into a mature follicle. With a combination of taking the testosterone (DHEA) and diet augmentation (insulin resistance plays a role) I was able to bring my AMH down enough to conceive. In short, AMH is a hugely important number. Know yours and keep getting it retested as it changes with your diet and lifestyle.

What are the causes of fertility?
The causes of infertility are different for males than females, and it's important to understand your specific issues so that you can develop a personalized care plan to combat them. In women, the most common causes of infertility include:

- Endometriosis
- PCOS
- Fallopian Tube Failures
- Fibroids
- Medications
- Sexually Transmitted Diseases
- Genetics
- Premature Ovarian Aging
- Hormonal Issues
- Autoimmune disease
- Ovulatory dysfunction
- Age

In males, common causes of infertility include:
- Structural abnormalities or damage to reproductive organs
- Abnormal or low sperm production
- Varicoceles
- Sexually transmitted diseases
- Environmental exposures

- Autoimmune disease
- Age

Endometriosis:

- There is some debate in the medical community if "mild" endometriosis affects infertility. I strongly believe that even when mild, endometriosis has an impact on fertility. More importantly, endometriosis impacts fertility negatively in many ways, though its impact on tubal function appears to be the most pressing. Investigations attempting to explain why patients with endometriosis often suffer from infertility have suggested that:
    - Their fallopian tubes may function abnormally, due to adhesion or scarring resulting from endometriosis invading the tubes (so-called tubal infertility)
    - Ovarian function may be adversely affected when endometriosis lesions invade the ovaries, possibly resulting in diminished ovarian reserve and sub-par egg quality
    - Endometriosis may release toxic substances which may harm embryos and/or their implantation capacity
    - Patients with endometriosis may be at a higher risk for miscarriages, lowering their live birth chances
    - Finally, there may be an immunological factor involved in endometriosis. Norbert Gleicher, MD, CHR's Medical Director and Chief Scientist, was the first to report on the possible association of autoimmunity and endometriosis, suggesting that endometriosis, indeed, may be an autoimmune disease. It is now widely accepted that the immune system, indeed, plays an important role in endometriosis-associated infertility

Polycystic Ovarian Syndrome:

Affecting about 6-12% of women in reproductive age, polycystic ovary syndrome (PCOS) is a "basket" of different medical conditions, with one finding in common: polycystic ovaries (PCO). In polycystic ovaries, multiple small cysts appear along the outer capsule of the ovaries on ultrasound imaging. PCOS is often associated with infertility, because of anovulation (lack of ovulation) and amenorrhea (lack of menstruation). However, with proper fertility treatments, PCOS patients can usually get pregnant with their own eggs. More on this in my PCOS handbook!

Premature Ovarian Aging:

Premature ovarian failure (POF), also known as primary ovarian insufficiency (POI), is a loss of ovarian function before the age of 40. POF can affect women at various ages, from their teenage years to their thirties. Women with POF are at a greater risk of a range of health issues, including osteoporosis, estrogen deficiency (hot flashes, vaginal dryness, etc.) and heart diseases.

These POF-related issues can usually be managed well with hormonal replacement. But for women with POF, fertility poses a challenge, as the loss of ovarian function means that the probability of pregnancy with their own eggs is greatly reduced.

Autoimmune Disease:

The term autoimmune disease refers to a varied group of more than 80 serious, chronic illnesses that involve almost every human organ system. In all these diseases, the body's immune system becomes misdirected, and attacks the very organs it was designed to protect. About 75% of autoimmune diseases occur in women, most frequently during the childbearing years. Women with autoimmune diseases experience miscarriage more often than other women and therefore require particular care in maintaining a pregnancy in addition to simply focusing on getting pregnant.

Autoimmune diseases can also affect connective tissue, the tissue that binds together various tissues and organs. It can also affect the nerves, muscles, endocrine system, and gastrointestinal system. There are many autoimmune diseases, with multiple sclerosis, Hashimoto's thyroiditis, rheumatoid arthritis being some of the most common.

Because abnormal immune function can affect fertility as well as miscarriage risk, affected women need two layers of treatment: a first layer to conceive, and a second to prevent pregnancy loss after conception. This is a very important point: it would not make sense to receive fertility treatment to get pregnant, only to experience an emotionally painful and potentially preventable pregnancy loss.

Ovulatory Dysfunction:

Ovulatory problems account for 20-30% of infertility cases. You can't get pregnant if you're not ovulating! Ovulation is a process of maturing eggs that have been "resting" in the ovaries since birth. Each day throughout a woman's life (until she reaches menopause), her eggs mature and move into an active state. Eggs are actually "active" in childhood as well, but there are no hormones to drive their development. Interesting, right? The hormones that come into play during puberty allow the activated eggs to mature, and at that point they compete with the other mature eggs to become the egg that will ovulate. After eggs commit to the maturation process, they either achieve successful ovulation or they die. Sounds harsh, especially when you consider that the aging ovary is the most common of ovulatory problems. In the 10 yrs prior to menopause, fewer and fewer eggs become present in the ovaries. When the remaining eggs fall below a critical level, cycles become irregular. Eggs that mature during the last decade of reproductive life are not as likely to establish a continuing pregnancy. For women who experience irregular cycles & ovarian aging, it may be necessary to use fertility medication to achieve ovulation.

In addition to hormonal issues like PCOS or an overactive pituitary gland, physical and mental stress can result in ovulatory problems (raise your hand if you're going to cut the next person to tell you *relax and it will happen*). It's not unusual for say, graduate school students to stop ovulating, although extreme weight loss, physical training/stress or even a deeply upsetting situation (like a death in the family) can all result in ovulatory problems. In many cases, this is temporary and normal cycling returns when the stressor is no longer present. In the case of extreme weight loss or exercise bulimia, an internist, reproductive endocrinologist and psychologist or psychiatrist are all often needed to correct the problem. Although it is possible to treat this type of anovulatory problem with fertility drugs, most medical professionals agree that it is safer and more effective to correct the underlying stressor.

Thyroid issues can also present as ovulatory concerns. If you have an underactive or overactive thyroid (hypo or hyperthyroidism), ovulatory problems may occur. Proper treatment of the thyroid abnormality will often restore regular ovulation.

Finally, there are some women who are born with ovaries that cannot produce eggs. Women with this condition cannot undergo puberty and usual have never had a period, although this is extremely rare.

The good news is that many ovulatory problems can be effectively treated, and once ovulation is restored, the chance of pregnancy returns to normal. Fortunately, today, the availability of egg donors can provide the opportunity for women with ovarian aging or abnormal ovarian development to achieve pregnancy.

Age:

Premature ovarian aging (POA) is defined as a younger woman having low or poor ovarian reserve relative to the expected reserve for her age. It is one of the major, most often overlooked causes of female infertility (that's what happened to me!) The ability of the ovaries to produce high quality eggs is known as Ovarian Reserve (OR). As women get older, their OR naturally declines as the number and quality of eggs decrease and it becomes harder to get pregnant. Women attempting pregnancy over age 40 often have trouble getting pregnant for this reason.

In approximately 10% of women, however, this decline of ovarian function occurs much earlier than normal. These women suffer from Premature Ovarian Aging (POA). Don't be confused if your provider refers to POA as 'occult primary ovarian insufficiency' or 'oPOI.' POA negatively impacts female fertility because smaller number of low-quality eggs make it more difficult to get pregnant. Once pregnant, the poor quality makes miscarriages more likely. Unfortunately, the quality of eggs decline in parallel with the quantity of eggs. Therefore, women with untreated diminished ovarian reserve experience the highest miscarriage rates of any IF diagnosis - approx. 95% of embryo quality comes from the egg, and poor-quality embryos are more likely to result in miscarriages.

Women with this condition have a hard time conceiving on their own, even with fertility treatments like IUI, if the treatment is not appropriate for their ovarian reserve status. But with appropriate care, like using DHEA and CoQ10 to enhance egg vitality or using aggressive ovarian stimulation protocols, women with this condition can conceive. So, take heart, mama!

The causes of premature ovarian aging are still unknown, although recent animal studies suggest that ovarian reserve is genetically controlled, and genetics is likely a factor (POA runs in families). If you are just starting on your infertility journey, be sure to check in with the women in your family to understand if they've had challenges with ovarian health.

Look at your medical history. Lifesaving procedures such as chemotherapy and radiation can cause premature ovarian aging (POA) or even premature ovarian failure (POF), which is why preserving fertility is recommended for young women with serious medical conditions that require these procedures. Surgeries involving the ovaries can also result in POA or POF when enough of the ovarian tissue is damaged/removed to reduce the ovary's ability to produce an egg.

As discussed previously, certain conditions (autoimmune disease, endometriosis, pelvic infections, tubal disease, etc.) can impact POA. Autoimmunity can be a downstream effect of POA when a patient's immune system attacks the ovaries. POA has also been associated with autoimmunity in general and a hyperactive immune system.

POA's Effects on Female Infertility:

- Leads to diminished ovarian reserve
- Poor response to ovarian stimulation in IVF cycles ("poor responder")
- Poor quality eggs
- Poor quality embryos
- Embryos with disproportionately high rate of chromosomal abnormalities (aneuploidy)
- Reduced number of euploid embryos (balanced set of chromosomes)
- Low pregnancy rates
- High miscarriage rates

When it comes to determining the pregnancy chances for each patient, it is important to distinguish between POA and POF (premature ovarian failure). While POF refers to a complete loss of the ovaries' ability to produce eggs, which makes pregnancy extremely difficult, patients with POA are still able to produce eggs, especially with specifically designed treatment.

Male Infertility:
As part of an initial infertility diagnostic workup, the fertility specialist often orders a semen analysis. Semen analysis tests the quantity and quality of the sperm. A complete semen analysis involves the assessment of many different factors, but the most important factors include:

- Motility- This term refers to how well the sperm moves. At least 50% of the sperm should 'swim' in a straight line; sperm that moves well is more likely to reach an egg.
- Morphology- This term refers to how the head of the sperm looks. At least 15% of the sperm should have a normal shape & structure with an oval shaped head. Abnormally shaped sperm are less likely to be able to fertilize an egg.
- Sperm Count- This figure refers to the number of sperm in a milliliter of semen. Sperm counts should be above 20 million in a milliliter of

sperm. A complete semen sample should have at least 40 million sperm.

When any one of these 3 factors are deemed abnormal, 'male infertility' may be diagnosed. But here's the real truth: no one really cares very much about sperm counts, motility and morphology as much as they want to understand how the sperm functions. Sperm has one biological function, which is to penetrate the wall of the egg (called the zona pellucida) to fertilize the egg. These factors are only approximations of that one crucial function of the sperm as there is ultimately no other reliable test to determine this function (ethics in testing live sperm against eggs is a challenge). Therefore, testing sperm function indirectly via a semen analysis is the next best thing. If all 3 factors are normal, sperm function will be normal as well (99% likelihood). If one or more parameters are abnormal, your physician will assume a fertilization problem exists. The severity of the problem is usually considered to be proportionate to the severity of the observed abnormality in the semen analysis.

My RE gave me a diagnosis of "Unexplained Infertility"...now what?
Hoo boy. This one must be one of the most frustrating diagnosis out there. Unexplained, huh? Great...let me get right on that. How are you supposed to solve for something if you don't even know what the root cause is? 15-20% of all infertility centers report a diagnosis of "unexplained infertility," while this is simply a 'garbage pail' diagnosis (and frankly a bit lazy if you ask me), many clinics don't look for subtle changes in the ways ovaries function and don't get picked up by routine testing. Sometimes there can be problems with embryos or implantation, or secondary immune factors that can be identified by immunologic testing. Perhaps what looks like a normal semen analysis with traditional criteria is actually causing your delay in conception, but you have to look deeper. Maybe you have an FSH higher than it should be or an AMH that is considered "normal" but is actually causing ovarian dysfunction (this was the case with me). In a recent longitudinal study by Oxford, 81% of couples with unexplained infertility achieved an ongoing pregnancy, and 74% of them were achieved spontaneously.

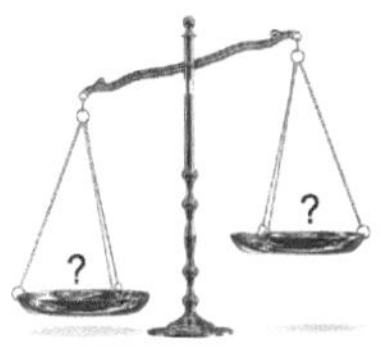

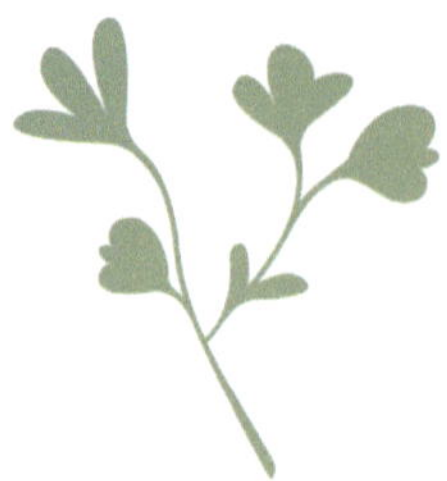

VI. Other Things No One Tells You

Just because 'lose weight' wasn't on your protocol from your RE, doesn't mean it's not important. Obviously, follow all the protocols and guides from your doctor, but know that there are other important factors at play to consider. Such as....

Thyroid & Insulin Resistance:

Ok, let's talk weight. Most Western doctors won't touch this topic with a 10-foot pole, but its critical to success in conception. Unfortunately, Western medicine teaches physicians to solve the problem, not the root cause of the issue, and your GYN or RE is simply not in the business of nutrition. If your weight is an issue for conception, no one is likely going to confront you about it. In addition to its being taboo, your physician is likely not a nutritionist. As a feminist, I don't think anyone should ever comment on the aesthetics of your physical body (positive or negatively). But if you are severely overweight and it's causing you to ovulate irregularly, that's going to be an issue until you get to a healthier weight as the hormones essential for conception live within your fat cells.

Alternatively, if you are underweight, it can be harder to get pregnant and maintain a successful pregnancy. No fat cells equals no baby. Now is not the time to lose 10 lbs.! And it's not just a numbers game.... just looking at your BMI ain't gonna cut it. You must have a body that is well nourished and healthy. Not only does this give you the best chances of conception, but it also gives you the best chance at a healthy baby! In my case, I was underweight for many years, which caused irregular menstrual cycles (compounded by my PCOS). Once I finally got serious about conceiving, I was at a healthy weight and even forced myself to stay 5-10lbs above what I thought looked "good" in jeans because I wanted better odds at conceiving. What I didn't know at the time, was that even though I had a healthy BMI on the heavier side, I was still malnourished. Malnourished? What? I live in the United States and I come from the suburbs! But given my undiagnosed celiac disease, with every molecule of gluten I ingested, the lining of my stomach and the filia blocked the absorption of the gluten to protect me...unfortunately it also blocked all the vitamins and minerals I should have been absorbing. So even at 5'2", 125lbs, I was still technically malnourished. Even if you don't have an underlying condition like celiac, if you are at a healthy weight, but your diet is candy bars and diet coke, your body is missing out on vital nutrients that form the basic building blocks of life.

Insulin resistance is a hot topic right now, particularly with the keto diet being as popular as it is. While there is a lot of research still ongoing, we know that 70% of all people experience some form of insulin resistance. If you're not following a modified paleo/keto/low carb low sugar diet, heavy in plants, you likely have this issue. More on diet & sample recipes in the Appendix (you gotta try Mr. Fertility Forest's kale....as someone who used to hate it, it's now my favorite vegetable....and baby Fertility Forest loves it as well!).

Does thyroid function play a role in infertility? How do I know if mine is an issue?

In addition to cleaning up your diet, make sure your thyroid function is being checked right off the bat. Your thyroid is a small butterfly-shaped gland in the base of your neck that produces hormones that travel throughout your body. Improper thyroid function has been linked to miscarriages and failures in embryo implantation. TSH stands for thyroid stimulating hormone. A TSH test is a blood test that measures this hormone. High TSH levels can mean your thyroid is not making enough thyroid hormones, a condition called hypothyroidism. Low TSH levels can mean your thyroid is making too much of the hormones, a condition called hyperthyroidism. A TSH test does not explain why TSH levels are too high or too low. If your test results are abnormal, your health care provider will probably order <u>additional tests</u> to determine the cause of your thyroid problem. These tests may include:

- T4 thyroid hormone tests

- T3 thyroid hormone tests

- Tests to diagnose Graves' disease, an autoimmune disease that causes hyperthyroidism

- Tests to diagnose Hashimoto's thyroiditis, an autoimmune disease that causes hypothyroidism

Normal ranges for thyroid tests may vary slightly among different laboratories, and typical ranges for common tests are given below. TSH normal values are 0.5 to 5.0 mIU/L. Make sure you confirm with your doctor as this should be a fasted test. Also, the research is still out on this, but researchers indicate that improving insulin resistance can have a positive impact on AMH. If your doctor doesn't order a TSH test for you, request one.

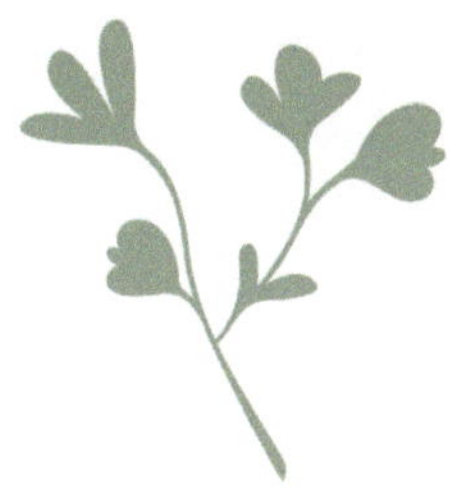

VII. Mental Treatment

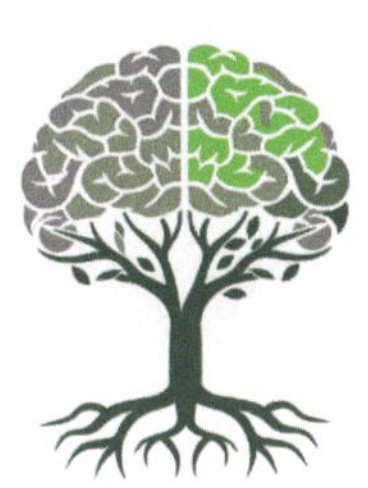

Studies have shown that women experiencing infertility have as high of levels of stress as people with terminal cancer. When a round of fertility treatments proves unsuccessful, women and couples can experience deep pain and grief. In fact, one study found that 50% of women and 15% of men cite infertility as the most upsetting experience of their lives (I know this was certainly up there for me!) Today, men are much more involved in the family and may feel a loss just as deeply. Although they do not experience the physical pain, the emotional pain can be just as real.

Women of color are more likely to experience infertility as compared to white women. However, women of color are also more likely to be blamed for their own infertility or have their emotional pain and valid medical concerns dismissed or ignored by physicians. In communities of color, there can be more importance placed on childbearing and being a strong mother who is naturally fertile. When a woman of color cannot fulfill that duty, it may be harder for her to seek treatment for infertility or mental health because she's not getting that support from her family.

And it's not just the infertility itself that's causing you distress. The hormone therapy many women need to treat the condition can have an impact on mental health. The hormones you are given will influence your mood, but it can be different for everyone. Look for signs such as: sleep disturbances, disruptions in libido, hot flashes, depression, and anxiety, among other symptoms. This was certainly the case for me; my doctor was confused when I told her how much I hated being on estrogen. For me, it caused a lot of brain fog, and I just didn't feel like myself. However, when I was put on testosterone, I felt great. I tend to be more competitive and aggressive than most females, and although my husband liked to joke that I was gonna start a bar fight, I finally felt like ME....and eventually ended up getting pregnant as a result.

Take note of your mental and emotional symptoms as well as physical throughout this process, and most importantly, HONOR those feelings. Don't dismiss them as they are important cues in your journey. Honor yourself by recognizing this is a difficult and emotional process, and don't be afraid to ask for help. There are multiple ways to get support. As your doctor if there are local support groups you can go to. For me, I made lifelong friendships with some of the women in my support group. I also saw a therapist; and if you can find one that specializes in infertility, all the better. Talk to your therapist or psychiatrist about how you feel and your medications. While some mental health medications are allowed during the infertility process, it's important to understand which are OK to use during your infertility journey and if you're already on medications, talk to your doctor about which you need to step down from.

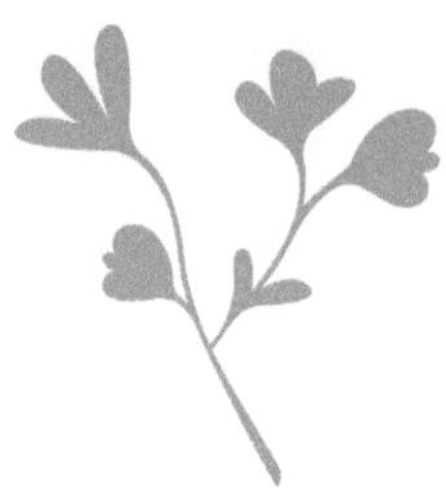

VIII. Important Conversations to Have with The People in Your Life

While infertility is common, there are a lot of people who haven't had any experience with it. As someone who is sensitized to it, you will likely encounter a lot of well meaning, but ignorant comments. And although they can be hurtful, I have found that the best responses are to use it as a teachable moment and educate the person or keep your responses brief. Below here are a few examples of how to talk to the important people in your life.

- Your spouse

Infertility is a lonely kind of pain. It can be difficult to have healthy & open conversations when you are feeling insecure and vulnerable. During this difficult time, you may find it helpful to have regular check-ins with your partner. Family planning is not a onetime conversation with your partner, just as opinions and preferences change over time, your feelings on infertility and family planning in general can change too. One of you may feel ready for certain treatments while the other may not. One of you may still want to keep trying, while the other is ready to crack. Additionally, infertility is not an inexpensive journey, so be open and check in frequently on the emotional as well as financial impacts of infertility.

Authentic, vulnerable conversation is the goal, and that begins with intentional questions. Use open ended questions, and if you're having trouble, write down your questions (start with 'how' what' or 'when') and take some time to process before sharing. It may take longer than you think but being intentional in your responses will go a long way towards healthy, vulnerable dialogue. Use "I" statements and communicate that you are in this together with your partner and you are a team. Make space for the negative emotions and don't sugarcoat it with your partner. Be honest about how you are feeling and don't minimize or ignore your feelings. Don't be afraid to share what you need right now from your partner. Even if what you have to say is painful in the moment, over time you'll both benefit from honest sharing. Be sure not to blame one partner or the other and remember that its crucial to reinforce the positive aspects of your relationship to reduce stress.

And if you find that things are getting too overwhelming, keep an open mind to getting professional help together. Couples thrive when they work through infertility as a team versus individuals. Don't be afraid to bring in some extra emotional support; therapy can be a safe place for couples to talk about how the dreams for the future you may look different now. Remember, getting outside help does not mean you've failed. It means you've succeeded in being honest and proactive. Most importantly, keep going. The first few conversations may be bumpy, and you may even feel like they were pointless. But if the two of you can be a team and support one another, this can be an experience you can grow from and deepen your relationship as you work to make your dreams of a family a reality.

- Relatives & Friends

When you're in the weeds of infertility, even the most well-meaning comment can put you over the edge. It's important to set clear boundaries with people that you care about so they know how to support you, as many are likely unfamiliar with the dynamics of infertility or how difficult it can truly be. Before moving forward with any conversations with people outside of your relationship, discuss with your partner how much detail you want to share or are comfortable sharing. I found that my husband, given his family culture, wanted to talk much more openly about our situation than I did. Pick a time to talk when people are not rushed or distracted and rehearse what you want to say. Words matter, so be sure you are communicating what you mean to convey.

Start with education. 1 in 8 couples, or 7 million people experience infertility. Let them know that infertility is a life crisis and how they can best support you. Explain that you may need a break from family gatherings, and that is about you and not them (particularly if you will be in a situation with new babies or young children). You can let them know that you will share results about a treatment or a procedure and ask them not to ask about pregnancy test or treatment results as that can cause more undue stress.

The hardest words to hear can be 'Guess what? I'm pregnant!" The best you can do is to share your happiness for your friend and if you choose, explain more fully why you are unable to celebrate wholeheartedly. Something like, "*I'm happy for you, but this is difficult news to hear when I am struggling with infertility. This is a really tough time for me, so please understand if I am unable to attend your shower or talk about the new baby. I wish you all the best of luck; I know you will be a fantastic mother."*

- Your boss

Once you've decided to pursue infertility treatment and learned a bit more about the standard of care with your physician, it will become obvious to you that you'll need some flexibility and collaboration with your employer to be able to execute your treatment plan. This can be intimidating, but it's critical that you advocate for yourself and set reasonable expectations between you and your boss. Pro tip: before you speak to your employer, have a plan in place. Be sure that you understand the treatment plan so that you can prepare for a work/life balance conversation with your boss. Be sure to understand what each step of the treatment plan entails, how often you'll need to be at the clinic, how much time visits typically take, and if there will need to be time off surrounding specific procedures. Be sure to consider the emotional impact during these procedures and do yourself a favor and don't overschedule yourself to give yourself buffer time in case you do react emotionally.

Be sure that you've researched your HR policies and benefits and think about the culture of your workplace when thinking about what you want to share and how you want the conversation to go. Drafting an outline for the conversation may be helpful, and as you do so, bear in mind the need to lead with the positive, be straightforward, illustrate your flexibility and commit to keeping lines of communication open.

Once you're ready to discuss, schedule time with your boss to discuss, ideally at a low stress time (Friday afternoons are great for this kind of discussion). Start by affirming your commitment to the organization and your dedication to the team's success. Let your boss know that you are facing a challenging time in your personal life that you are working to balance with your professional responsibilities. Assure your boss that you will be diligent and flexible in both work responsibilities and attention to your medical care. Emphasize that while what you've surfaced represents the currently proposed treatment plan, things may change, and you'll need the margin to adapt to the inevitable changes in any infertility journey. Consider following up the conversation with a brief thank you note for their time and consideration of your circumstances.

How much you share and how specific you are is totally up to your discretion. But some things to consider should include company culture, your relationship with your boss, your level of seniority and the intensity or evasiveness of the treatment you expect to undergo.

When talking with your employer at your infertility treatment, keep the conversation simple & straightforward. This is a medical condition, so treat it as such. Protect the information or the emotions that are too private for you to share comfortable. While you can be honest that this is a painful and challenging experience, try to maintain your composure as you want to remain professional and do not want to make things uncomfortable.

When sharing your treatment plan, explain how you anticipate the schedule will impact your day to day, projects, and productivity. Commit to keeping your boss in the loop on any issues the treatments may have on your workload. Ask your employer on his or her preference for sharing this information with your co-workers. Collaborating with your boss on this issue will pave the way for smoother communication when flex schedules or responsibilities may be e. It also allows you to have a say in how much or little is shared regarding your personal situation.

Consider a sit down with your Human Resources manager if you are accessing your employee benefits to cover your infertility treatment. Be sure that you understand your policy and how to maximize your benefits. Understand your company's Americans with Disabilities Act, Family Medical Leave (FMLA) policy. For example, some companies do not offer 'sick time' anymore, so it's helpful to understand how to manage time off when its needed.

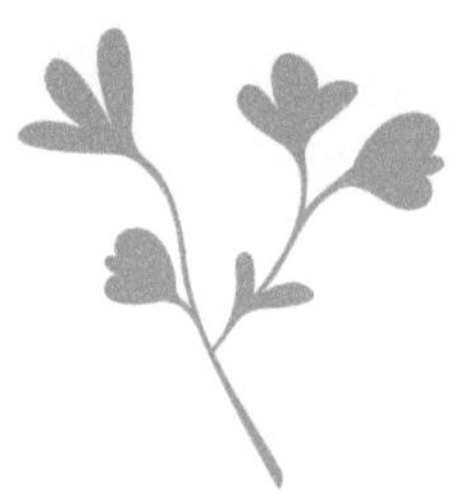

IX.   Conclusion:

Infertility can be a long and lonely road, but it doesn't have to be that way. By approaching things with an attitude of advocacy, tenacity and radical vulnerability you can make it through successfully, with thriving personal relationships, a feeling of investment in yourself and your health and most importantly, a beautiful baby in your arms. Just because you were told no doesn't mean you take no for an answer. Understand that your providers are operating with a framework; and if that framework doesn't work for you, don't be afraid to bust out of it and find one that DOES work. If you need more support, join our community on Facebook or Instagram where we have regular support meetings, protocol updates, recipes, best practices, tips and more. Yes, being stuck in the weeds of infertility is a challenge, but your support team at Fertility Forest is here to help you find the way out and into the family of your dreams. Take heart, mama. You got this.

www.ingramcontent.com/pod-product-compliance
Lightning Source LLC
Chambersburg PA
CBHW040250240726
48664CB00001B/337